APPLE CIDER VINEGAR

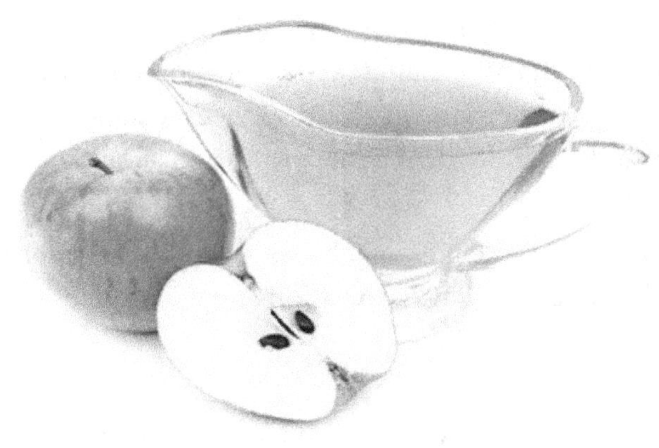

By Julia Bond

Copyright © 2017 by Julia Bond

The trademarks that are used are without any consent, and the publication of the trademark is without permission or backing by the trademark owner. All trademarks and brands within this book are for clarifying purposes only and are the owned by the owners themselves, not affiliated with this document.

Disclaimer and Terms of Use: The Author and Publisher has strived to be as accurate and complete as possible in the creation of this book, notwithstanding the fact that he does not warrant or represent at any time that the contents within are accurate due to the rapidly changing nature of the Internet. While all attempts have been made to verify information provided in this publication, the Author and Publisher assumes no responsibility for errors, omissions, or contrary interpretation of the subject matter herein.

Any perceived slights of specific persons, peoples, or organizations are unintentional. In practical advice books, like anything else in life, there are no guarantees of results. Readers are cautioned to rely on their own judgment about their individual circumstances and act accordingly.

This book is not intended for use as a source of legal, medical, business, accounting or financial advice. All readers are advised to seek services of competent professionals in the legal, medical, business, accounting, and finance fields.

TABLE OF CONTENTS

INTRODUCTION

Apple cider vinegar is perhaps the number one natural remedy chronicled throughout human history. The use of vinegar as a tonic has been documented as far back as 5000 BC by the Babylonians who were using the date palm to make wine and vinegar.

They used it as a food and for a pickling agent. Vinegar residues have been found in ancient Egyptian urns dated 3000 BC. Chinese historical documents from 1200 BC tout the glories of vinegar benefits as well.

The reasons for its popular medicinal use and as an energizing drink are scientifically well founded by modern science also. Apple cider vinegar benefits are a result of its source - the noble apple - famous for the saying An apple a day keeps the doctor away.

Apples contain not only vitamins, minerals, and antioxidants, but also dietary fiber. In addition they contain virtually no fat or sodium.

All of the apples goodness is miraculously transferred to apple cider vinegar especially when it's left untouched or in other words unprocessed.

Apple cider vinegar made from whole apples and not pasteurized or filtered contains not only all of the apples nutrients but also many additional enzymes and organic acids produced during the two fermentations required to turn apples into vinegar.

The long list of apple cider benefits range from an antiseptic to an antioxidant while providing a host of absorbable minerals such as potassium and magnesium including pectin, and a water soluble fiber, which is one of the many reasons for the success of the cider vinegar diet.

The recommended method of using apple cider vinegar is to make it into a tonic by mixing 2 or 3 teaspoons of ACV in an 8 ounce glass of water and drinking it before or during each meal.

One point to remember when taking apple cider vinegar between meals or before going to bed is to always rinse your mouth to avoid any prolonged vinegar contact with the enamel on your teeth.

Another way of dealing with this minor setback is to mix a tsp. of baking soda in the vinegar before you add water. It is always fun to watch it fizz up! Besides the added alkalinity provided by the baking soda is a definite health plus.

As far as ACV remedies are concerned the list literally ranges from A to Z. It starts at acne and asthma and runs to warts and weight loss ending with yeast infections including such ailments as cancer, eczema, fatigue, fungus, headaches, heartburn, insomnia, sore throat, ulcers, and varicose veins in between - to list just a few.

In short, apple cider vinegar lives up to its reputation of being the simplest answer to perfect health and a timeless cure all as well. A prize in any persons natural remedy medicine chest and a powerful preventative to whatever ails, not to forget its age old popularity as a world class tonic.

Make sure you always use pure unprocessed organic apple cider vinegar with the mother still in it, and you can rely on its amazing properties to help provide you and your family with a long and healthy life.

This GUIDE has been fully packaged with many wonders ACV has to offer.

LET'S DIVE IN!

CHAPTER 1: A GOOD DRINK FOR YOUR HEALTH

Everyone is familiar with the old saying-an apple each day keeps the physician away. Apples are produced into a type of vinegar. Several studies have disclosed the great apple cider vinegar advantages.

While these had already been recognized even prior to, the advantages had been not given significance. Some people just consider of it as a kitchen condiment.

You might have noticed numerous publications that tout the several benefits of apple cider vinegar. So what precisely is vinegar and how is it very good for you? It is made when apples are crushed into a mixture of juices and pulp; this is allowed to ferment until an acetic acid is made.

Probably the most well-liked uses for this wealthy vinegar supplement will be the weight reduction. Several folks swear that you simply can drop pounds steadily just by taking two tablespoons of this nectar each and every day. This will be the only requirement for the diet plan. Just take the vinegar and you might be nicely on your way to a slimmer form.

No clear explanation is offered as to how does it aid in weight reduction, but people who have utilized this vinegar say that they did lose a considerable quantity of weight which they think was the result of standard consumption of vinegar.

It can be largely believed that the vitamins, minerals, enzymes and amino acids increase our metabolism at the same time as suppress appetite naturally. Hence, the effectiveness of apple cider for weight reduction got popularized.

It is possible to use the apple cider vinegar as home remedies for numerous illnesses. One belief is its anti-aging properties. It performs detoxification and cleansing functions, which result to body detox.

As a healing elixir, it possesses normal antibiotics and antiseptics which are employed by the body to combat bacteria and germs within the human program, explicitly within the digestive tract. It's also helpful to the digestive program because it breaks down the proteins, fats and minerals from the food you eat.

You'll be able to get the apple cider vinegar rewards if it's taken every day. You are able to use it as a salad dressing or a marinade. You may also buy it in capsule form. If you would like homemade apple cider vinegar, you'll find some issues which you need to bear in mind for the vinegar to be useful.

There are many actions which you need to follow, and you ought to not use metal container or aluminum. It is possible to make this mixture in glass, wood, plastic, enamel and stainless steel. You need to not miss out on following each and every step which includes fermentation for you to create vinegar successfully.

CHAPTER 2: HEALTH BENEFITS OF APPLE CIDER VINEGAR

Apple cider vinegar (ACV) has been called a cure for everything. Health enthusiasts have used it for everything from acne and allergies to sore throats and warts. Vinegar in its many forms has been used for centuries for all sorts of folk remedies.

Recently with the flood of people turning to home and natural based remedies, apple cider vinegar has come to light as an especially useful health tonic.

People are often skeptical about something as common as apple cider vinegar being such an effective treatment for so many ailments. Folk remedy experts have long used it as a natural cure-all.

When you think of apple cider, you probably think of fall. A warm sweet glass full of apples and spice that warms the body on a cool fall day and this delicious drink is where this miracle tonic gets its start.

It begins life as apples that are pulverized to make cider. This cider is then combined with yeast which turns the sugars in the cider into alcohol. From this point, the cider wine continues to ferment until it sours and turns into vinegar.

ACV HAS MANY CLAIMS TO FAME INCLUDING:

- A natural acne fighter and skin toner

- A wart remover

- A hair rinse to brighten and nourish dull hair

- Removes lice, fleas, ticks, etc

- Cures infections

- Removes toxins

- A natural aftershave

- Relieves sunburn

- And so much more!

The most important benefits of using apple cider vinegar are the effects that take place inside of the body. When added to your daily diet, its effects are pretty amazing. Let's take a look at a few of these benefits:

IMPROVED DIGESTION AND WEIGHT LOSS

ACV can help restore normal acid levels in your digestive system which helps break down fats and proteins. This allows your body to digest food easier and more thoroughly which promotes nutrient absorption by the body and overall health.

Apple cider vinegar can also help you feel fuller which will help you eat less and take some of the strain off of your digestive system.

It is also been shown to help regulate blood sugar levels which promotes weight loss and lowers the risk of diabetes. One study also showed that regular supplementation with apple cider vinegar reduced body fat, triglyceride levels, and was effective for overall weight loss. It is a great weight loss supplement and an easy way to fight obesity.

HELPS PREVENT CANCER

Apple cider vinegar slows the growth of cancer cells and possibly even kills cancer cells. The results of studies have been somewhat contradictory on this subject but many possibilities are mentioned. Some think that the acetic acid in vinegar could be the cancer fighting ingredient.

Others have proposed the pectin found in apples as well as polyphenols as possible anti-cancer ingredients. The true source is still a mystery but preliminary evidence has shown that apple cider vinegar is useful in the prevention of some forms of cancer.

IMPROVED CHOLESTEROL LEVELS AND BLOOD PRESSURE

A preliminary study performed in rats has shown that apple cider vinegar can significantly reduce cholesterol in the body. Since the study was performed on rats, some speculate that these properties may not be the same in humans. Further studies are needed to confirm but preliminary evidence is positive.

A similar study also showed positive results for lowering of blood pressure and heart disease as well. Due to the low number of side effects and the evidence suggesting it may reduce overall risk factors for heart disease, a regular dose of apple cider vinegar might be good advice.

LIVER AND OTHER ORGAN DETOXIFICATION

The anti-bacterial properties of apple cider vinegar help cleanse the body of toxin build-up as well as reduce levels of harmful bacteria. The body's PH balance is also stabilized by regular doses as well which helps to promote the natural cleansing effect of the body.

Apple cider vinegar has also been used to treat allergies as well by cleansing mucous out of the sinuses and cleansing the lymph nodes.

When considering taking apple cider vinegar, make sure to find organic, unfiltered, and unpasteurized vinegar. You want untreated vinegar to maximize the health properties.

Before beginning any supplement program, even a natural one, speak with your doctor about possible side effects and interactions with any medications you are taking. Apple cider vinegar can be taken straight from the bottle or through other forms such as pills to avoid the sour taste and acidity.

CHAPTER 3: HOW TO USE APPLE CIDER VINEGAR FOR WEIGHT LOSS

Apple cider vinegar is prepared by the fermentation of apple juice. It is a natural remedy for a variety of health issues and has been resorted to for years.

It has a lot to offer when it comes to weight loss- helps break down the complex fats and carbohydrates; reduces blood sugar level and cholesterol; reduces the food cravings; aids in digestion and body detox.

It is a low-calorie natural supplement with various nutrients and active ingredients- minerals, vitamins, soluble fibers, antioxidants and natural acids and enzymes- that helps to deal with obesity.

It is prudent to know that apple cider vinegar in its concentrated (undiluted) form is a strong acid that should never be consumed raw. Our esophagus tube (food pipe) is not equipped to handle the same and can get severely damaged.

Hence, it makes sense to dilute it with water so that the intensity comes down. Also, it is important to monitor the dosage regularly. Start with 5-10 ml per day and gradually increase it up to 30 ml (2 tablespoons) per day. Going beyond 30 ml is generally not recommended.

Let us discuss how Apple Cider Vinegar will help you to lose some weight and change your life for good:

• HELPS TO REDUCE CHOLESTEROL LEVEL

Bile is a viscous yellowish liquid produced by the liver that helps to break down the dietary fats and to dispose off the leftover cholesterol and other toxins from the liver. Poor bile production hampers the liver activity which may result in accumulation of fats and cholesterol to cause obesity.

Consuming one tablespoon of apple cider vinegar early in the morning kick-starts the bile production to promote fat breakdown and cholesterol decomposition.

• LOWERS THE BLOOD SUGAR LEVEL

A spike in the blood sugar level increases the cravings for snacks and unhealthy processed foods which is a big turn off if you are trying to shed a few pounds.

• AIDS IN BLOCKING CARBOHYDRATES (STARCH)

Gone are the days, when it was believed that carbohydrates are bad for health. The new age of dieticians recommends consumption of carbohydrates on a regular basis to ensure a balanced diet.

The starch contained in carbohydrates has a tendency to quickly convert into glucose and stimulate the release of insulin in the body. The insulin triggers the storage of glucose in the form of fat. Hence, eating starchy food pushes your body into the fat storage mode.

HOW IS APPLE CIDER VINEGAR GOING TO HELP HERE?

The acetic acid content in the vinegar interferes with the body's ability to digest starch. It helps to reduce the storage of glucose in the form of fat. Over a period of time, this starch blockage activity would definitely have an effect on the body weight.

• PROMOTES A HEALTHY DIGESTIVE SYSTEM

Your gut contains trillions of probiotics (healthy bacteria) that helps to breakdown the complex food particles; combat the growth of disease causing microbes and regulates the immune system.

Apple cider vinegar acts as a catalyst for these probiotics. The probiotics feed on the pectins contained in apple cider vinegar for growth and development. Hence, apple cider vinegar helps to maintain an optimum gut flora for smooth digestion and body metabolism.

• SUPPRESSES THE APPETITE

Apple cider vinegar contains pectins- a type of soluble fibers which provides a feeling of fullness to suppress the appetite for all the good reasons.

• IT ACTS AS A MILD LAXATIVE AND DIURETIC IN NATURE

Apple cider vinegar acts as a mild laxative to accelerate the elimination process and ensure regular bowel movements. Also, it has a diuretic effect to release the excess stored water from the body.

• PROMOTE BODY DETOX

Body detoxification refers to the thorough cleansing of the body to get rid of accumulated body wastes- undigested food, cholesterol, saturated fats and disease causing microbes. Due to unhealthy diet and poor lifestyle habits, the body metabolism gets slow down and piling up of body toxins starts.

The combined effect of the sluggish body metabolism and accumulated body toxins would result in obesity. Apple cider vinegar is a detoxifying elixir- natural and safe. It promotes digestion, speed up the body metabolism, relieves constipation and excretes excess water from your body to detoxify your body from inside.

HOW TO CONSUME APPLE CIDER VINEGAR

Add 1-2 teaspoon (5-10 ml) of raw apple cider vinegar in one glass (250 ml) of water, stir well and drink it before the meals. If it causes temporary heartburn or irritation, simply dilute it with more water. You may mix it with your juice or other beverages as well. Some people prefer to sprinkle over the salads and other food preparations as per their taste.

The maximum, optimum dosage per day is 30 ml.

PRECAUTIONARY MEASURES AND POSSIBLE SIDE EFFECTS

In general, apple cider vinegar is a natural, safe drink for people of all ages. Do consider below safety measures to get the best benefits:

- Avoid drinking it as the first thing in the morning- empty stomach- as it may irritate the gut lining and cause burning sensation.

- Dilute it enough- one teaspoon in one glass of water seems a good ratio.

- Due to acid content, over consumption of apple cider vinegar can damage the esophagus tube and tissues. Also, it can cause hypokalemia- a condition when the potassium in the blood falls below the required level.

- Don't forget to rinse your mouth well after drinking apple cider vinegar otherwise the acid in vinegar can erode the tooth enamel. Also, it can cause yellow staining on the teeth.

- During the initial few days of consumption, you may experience temporary symptoms such as diarrhea, stomach cramp, heartburn or headache. In majority of the cases, these symptoms would fade away within a few days. If the symptoms persist, stop consuming it and discuss with a health expert

- Pregnant ladies, nursing women and people with chronic health conditions should consult their doctors before consuming it.

In short, start slow- with small quantity and gradually increase it up to 2 tablespoons a day in well diluted form for optimum results.

Benefits of apple cider vinegar for weight loss are obvious. But, being a natural remedy, it should not be considered as a miracle and it would bring the best results when combined with a healthy, low-calorie diet and positive lifestyle with regular physical workout.

CHAPTER 3: APPLE CIDER VINEGAR FLU REMEDY

Apple cider vinegar has been used to treat various illnesses for centuries. If one can get past its bitter taste, one can find relief in its healing attributes.

One of its more common purposes is to stave off a cold or flu. It is said to help cure a sore throat, soothe a stubborn cough, and treat a sinus infection, the usual symptoms that accompany a cold or flu. Using an apple cider vinegar flu remedy is easy, natural, and safe for most individuals.

HOW IT WORKS

When you contract a cold, your body's pH factor becomes slightly more alkaline. Apple cider vinegar, which is acidic, helps to rebalance the body's acid level.

SINUS INFECTION

In the case of a sinus infection, the apple cider vinegar remedy slows down mucus production and most often eliminates watery eyes because it contains high amounts of potassium.

It will rapidly thin the mucous, turning it from thick green or white to clear and runny. Apple cider vinegar contains many vitamins, nutrients and trace elements of copper, iron, silicon, magnesium, phosphorous, and calcium.

HOW TO TAKE IT

There are several ways to integrate apple cider vinegar into your diet in order to benefit from its remedial effects. The degree of effectiveness of an apple cider vinegar flu remedy is not solely based on how you take it, but also on when you take it. Some use it as a daily tonic, while others ingest it at the very first sign of a cold or sinus infection.

Since the taste is bitter, it is often mixed with other liquids. You can dilute 1/8 to 1/4 cup of apple cider vinegar into 16 ounces of water or juice, and sip the drink throughout the day.

If you are the brave type, dilute 2 tablespoons of apple cider vinegar into 8 ounces of water or juice and drink it all at once, 3 times per day.

When added to apple juice, it tastes like cider and is much more pleasant to drink.

It can also be stirred into a cup of tea.

If drinking apple cider vinegar is out of the question, add it to various sauces, marinades, and/or dressings.

The recommended dosage for apple cider vinegar is up to 3 tablespoons daily. It is also available in capsule form at many health food and vitamin stores. Taking a capsule every day keeps your body's pH level stable, rendering your immune system strong to fight off a cold or flu.

OTHER REMEDIAL USES FOR APPLE CIDER VINEGAR FLU

To help relieve chest congestion due to a cold or flu, soak a piece of brown paper in apple cider vinegar and cover one side with black pepper. Strap the paper (pepper-side down) to the chest area and leave on for approximately 30 minutes.

To calm a stubborn cough due to a cold or flu, sprinkle some apple cider vinegar onto the pillow before you sleep.

To soothe a sore throat due to a cold or flu, mix equal parts of apple cider vinegar and water and gargle every hour, making sure to rinse your mouth thoroughly afterwards in order to prevent the acid from eroding the enamel on your teeth.

To relieve a sinus headache and stuffy nose, add 1/8 of a cup of apple cider vinegar to the water solution in the vaporizer.

CHAPTER 4: APPLE CIDER VINEGAR BENEFITS FOR BEAUTY

Apple cider vinegar, sometimes referred to as cider vinegar or ACV, is made from cider or apple must. It has become very popular because of its many health benefits and beauty properties.

Because of it high potassium content, it is best to consult with a health care professional before taking ACV. Although you can make your own apple cider vinegar, you can find it in a natural state at any health food store. Let's explore some of the benefits of apple cider vinegar.

HOW TO USE APPLE CIDER VINEGAR

Apple cider vinegar can promote healthier skin and hair as well as be beneficial for health. For more specific ways in which apple cider can help treat specific ailments, contact a nutritionist who will be better equipped to answer specific questions. For more general uses, you can try apple cider vinegar in some of the following ways.

INTERNAL USE

Research has shown that ACV can assist the body in its daily functions as well as fight off colds and influenza. It helps in digestion, lowers bad cholesterol, strengthens the heart, lowers blood pressure and stabilizes blood sugar. It also contains anti-oxidants that help fight some types of cancer. It can cure an upset stomach by drinking it as a daily tonic.

To make your own daily tonic, mix equal parts of apple cider vinegar and honey in a glass of water. Usually, one tablespoon of ACV and one tablespoon of honey in 8 ounces of warm or cold water would be a general guideline, but feel free to tweak this recipe depending on your personal preferences.

There are also other ways to drink it. You could add it to apple juice or add a bit of fresh cinnamon to neutralize its taste (some coffee shops serve apple cider with a cinnamon stick).

EXTERNAL USE

If your feet feel tired and ache, give them a bath. Put half a cup of apple cider vinegar in a tub of warm water. Wiggle your toes around and let your feet soak for a few minutes. A footbath is a great way to relax before heading off to bed.

If your body is too acidic, take a vinegar bath. To properly restore the acid to alkaline balance in your body, simply add 1 to 2 cups of apple cider vinegar to a warm bath. Soak your body for about 45 minutes. Aside from clearing your body from excess acid, a vinegar bath helps anyone with a dry or irritated skin make it feel soft.

If baths aren't your thing, consider mixing one cup each of ACV and warm water in a spray bottle. After your shower, spray your entire body with the mixture. Wait a few minutes and rinse. Your whole body will feel refreshed.

Other benefits of apple cider vinegar include it's topically use on different body parts, especially the face. For a deep cleansing steam face wash, add 3 tablespoons of ACV to a pan of boiled water and lean your face over it.

Cover your head with a towel for a few minutes to allow the steam to open up your pores and loosen any impurities from your skin's surface.

COMMERCIAL PRODUCTS ON THE MARKET

Aside from the natural form of apple cider vinegar, many commercial products also exist. Such products include body washes and hair and facial products. Taking ACV in its natural state is just as beneficial if not better than these products.

Because apple cider vinegar is very acidic, never drink it straight. Always dilute it with water. After drinking ACV, you should rinse your mouth with water. Also, do not brush your teeth right away because it might grind the vinegar into your enamel.

A great way to avoid ACV touching your teeth is to drink it with a straw. ACV tablets are a great alternative to the liquid, although they don't work as fast. Also, avoid eye contact with apple cider vinegar as the acid will burn and redden the eyes

The benefits of apple cider vinegar seem endless. These simple methods and ways of using ACV are all great and inexpensive. More importantly, they have proven methods beneficial to your body and to the environment. As long as you use it carefully and for recognized, healthy purposes, apple cider vinegar benefits will continue to reveal themselves.

CHAPTER 5: HOW TO USE APPLE CIDER VINEGAR TO CURE ACNE

Apple Cider Vinegar otherwise known as (ACV) is an effective natural bacteria fighting agent that has many elements such as calcium, potassium, magnesium, chlorine, sodium, iron, sulfur and etc.

All these elements are vital for a healthy body especially to promote healthy skin development. These anti-bacterial properties make it a good topical home remedy for acne.

The main ingredient of ACV is acetic acid. It helps to exfoliate the dead skin cells gently, kills the bacteria propionibacterium acnes which is generally known as P-acnes and neutralizes the sebum which is the oily substance P-acnes feeds and thrives on.

HOW IS APPLE CIDER VINEGAR MADE?

Apple cider vinegar is obtained by the fermentation of apple cider or apple must which is made from crushed organic apples. Just for your information, fermentation means an act of conversion.

Organic apples have some kind of bacteria and yeast on their skins. So when they are crushed, you get pure apple juice with a mixture of bacteria and yeast.

After which you leave it to mature for a while. During this process, sugar in the apple cider is broken down by yeast and bacteria which turns into alcohol. It's more like a brewing process which eventually turns into vinegar after a second fermentation.

If you don't have all the time or resources to make one at home, you can easily purchase ACV from any departmental stores. First of all, make sure you get the organic ACV with the labels saying 'With the Mother' with an ideal acidity (pH) level of five to seven.

This means that it is in raw and pure form characterized by dark, cloudy, web-like bacterial foam which is brownish in color.

BENEFITS OF APPLE CIDER VINEGAR FOR YOUR SKIN

ACV contains acids one of which is alpha-hydroxy acid which have been extracted directly from the apples. These acids help dissolve the oil and sebum that clogs the pores and eventually un-clogs them. This will encourage skin renewal.

It is known to cure allergies from pets, food and environmental pollution, high cholesterol, flu, chronic fatigue, sinus infections, sore throats, arthritis and gout just to name a few.

However its most popular benefit is associated with weight loss. ACV is known to break down fat and that a daily dose of apple cider vinegar in water helps to keep high blood pressure in control within just two weeks.

It also helps to regulate the pH of your skin by simply diluting it with two parts of water and spreading the concoction over your face using a cotton ball as a toner overnight and washing it off the next morning. Please be mindful that you dilute it with larger portions of water since you are going to leave it on your skin for long hours.

It also helps to lighten age spots by dabbing ACV directly on them for about twenty minutes or so daily depending on the size of them. Besides it also helps to cleanse your liver by getting rid of accumulated toxins and recharging its efficiency.

HOW TO USE APPLE CIDER VINEGAR FOR ACNE?

The usage of this varies with the severity of your acne. Most of the time, users dilute it with water and apply it with a cotton ball over their spots as it seems to work very well. ACV is considered a good replacement for antibiotics as it helps to treat bacterial infections.

You can probably use apple cider vinegar in two ways; one as an internal tonic and as topical antibacterial solution.

Follow these steps and you might see some considerable results. First take three table spoons of ACV to a bottle of water and mix them well thoroughly. Then apply it on your face with a cotton ball as an astringent.

Try using three different cotton balls on your face. Use one for your forehead, another for your cheeks and nose and one for your chin. If you happen to have an oily nose in particular, use a separate one for that.

This is to prevent spreading bacteria from one place to all over your face which eventually would cause more breakouts on other areas of your face. Though this is quite uncommon, it's better to be safe than sorry.

Leave it for about ten to fifteen minutes and rinse it thoroughly with warm water. Then use a soft clean towel to pat your skin dry. Repeat this procedure three times a day for maximum effect.

For those who have severe forms of acne infection, you can apply lower dosage of ACV diluted with three to four parts of water and leave it overnight to do its job and wash it off the next day with warm water.

Remember that you use lower strength of ACV should you want to apply and leave it on your skin for longer periods.

Another thing you can do is to drink it with water with a few table spoons as a tonic every morning. This helps to prevent acne breakouts, reduce infection and dry out inflammations. The only thing you need to be aware of is that it might not taste pleasant at all. Just try drinking it like water and you will be fine.

If you have some really bothersome prominent pimples, I would recommend mixing one part of ACV with three parts of water and dab it onto the pimple. Leave it there for about fifteen minutes and wash it off with warm water.

SOME TIPS AND WARNINGS

Never attempt to apply full-strength ACV on the face as there have been reported cases of skin damage, irritations and burns. So be cautious about using this remedy especially for those who have sensitive skin.

Always use raw, unfiltered and unpasteurized apple cider vinegar. This will give you the best results.

After using apple cider vinegar, dab some tea tree oil on your acne. Tea tree oil works wonders for healing skin.

If you are allergic to apples, then apple cider vinegar is not for you.

Do not use in combination with other acne medications. This will lead to complications and over-drying of the skin.

When you are applying ACV, it is best to start out with the weakest combinations of four parts of water to it. If you are comfortable with it, then work up to stronger mixtures. That means reducing the amount of water.

Tingling sensations are pretty normal while using ACV, but if you start experiencing some burning sensations, rinse it off immediately with cold water.

Everything about apple cider vinegar has been pretty positive except for the astringency of the vinegar which you must take caution of when applying it on your face. I would recommend starting with a lower dosage of it and then moderate it to higher strength as you keep adapting to the topical solution.

It's normal to feel any tingling sensation as it is an indication that it's working. However if you start experiencing any burning effects then wash it off immediately and lower the strength of ACV.

For better results, use a water-based skin moisturizer to apply on your skin after each ACV treatment. This is to prevent your skin from getting too dehydrated due to the astringent characteristics of ACV.

I would like to point out that even though apple cider vinegar can remove some surface bacteria on the skin, it is not a long-term solution that can truly attack acne at its root. There are just about many causes of acne and bacteria are one of them.

It's more or less suitable for those who have mild to moderate acne and could see results in just a couple of weeks. For severe cases, it could really take a long time to heal it. Have patience and you will rule the world! The good thing is that you are doing it naturally and definitely not burning your pockets in the process.

It all makes sense to try out this inexpensive home remedy before switching to more expensive products. Even if you need to, the severity of your acne condition would have improved and you wouldn't have to spend a long time undergoing any medical procedures laid down for you by any dermatologist.

CHAPTER 6: GET RID OF DANDRUFF WITH APPLE CIDER VINEGAR

If you suffer from dandruff, you know how itchy and annoying it can be. It may feel like there is no product out there that will treat dandruff because you have tried to find it. What if the solution was not found in the medicine aisle?

Instead, it may be sitting on your grocery store shelf. You can get rid of dandruff with apple cider vinegar. You may wonder how something so acidic can actually be used on your scalp. If you are tired of suffering from the itching get rid of dandruff with apple cider vinegar.

Dandruff is white flakes found on the scalp. It usually does not cause any additional problems besides the uncomfortable itching. There could be different reasons for dandruff to develop; stress, imbalanced hormones, illness, medication, elevated oil production in the body, and more.

When the scalp becomes inflamed even slightly, it can cause dead skin cells to produce. Once the oil in the scalp combine with the dead skin cells, it will form a cluster of dandruff. Now you can get rid of dandruff with apple cider vinegar and find instant relief.

Now that you know what causes dandruff, you can begin to treat it more effectively. You can get rid of dandruff with apple cider vinegar. The apple cider vinegar will help replace the pH balance on the scalp.

In addition, it can also provide a shine to your hair that shampoo cannot give you. The best way to heal something is to restore and replace what it is missing so it will balance itself out. The body was designed to heal itself.

To get rid of dandruff with apple cider vinegar, you first need to shampoo your hair with a mild shampoo. Don't worry about stocking up on a dandruff shampoo because you won't need it.

These shampoos are expensive and they don't always cure the problem. The vinegar that you use will provide everything your scalp needs. Once you have rinsed your hair you are ready to add the vinegar solution.

You want to combine a mixture of apple cider vinegar and warm water. That will be two parts of the apple vinegar to one part of the warm water.

If your dandruff is very hard to treat and the mixture is not working right away, you may want to try a stronger combination and add more vinegar and less water. And this is how you get rid of dandruff with apple cider vinegar.

For an effective way to get rid of dandruff with apple cider vinegar, pour the vinegar and warm water mixture over wet rinsed hair. You can also place it in a spray bottle and spray it on so you know that you are reaching all the areas of the scalp.

The smell of apple cider vinegar is a bit strong so you may want to rinse it out but it is not necessary to do so unless you cannot tolerate the smell.

You should begin to see results shortly after beginning the treatment.

CHAPTER 7: YEAST INFECTION

Anybody who has ever had a yeast infection knows that they are not fun to have. Luckily for us, apple cider vinegar actually works as an effective home remedy for relief. When used correctly, it can actually help you to get relief from those nasty symptoms.

If you are a woman, you might be experiencing itching or burning, swelling, redness, and pain. If you are a man, you may be experiencing, swelling, red dots, dry skin, peeling skin, pain, or burning. If this is the case for you, then apple cider vinegar is a great way to get relief from some of these symptoms.

In this chapter, I want to tell you exactly how you can use apple cider vinegar to get relief from your yeast infection. If this home remedy doesn't give you relief, you can always try many of the other home remedies available.

There are actually 2 different ways you can use apple cider vinegar to get relief from your yeast infection. I would like to discuss each method with you now.

1. BATH + A.C.V.

One of the easiest ways to get relief from your yeast infection is by taking a bath. I know someone who said a bath helped them tremendously, but adding apple cider vinegar to the mix will be even more beneficial.

All you have to do is add 2 cups of apple cider vinegar to a warm bath, stir, and lay in the mixture for 15 minutes. After your bath, dry off, and put on cotton underwear afterward, preferably.

2. A.C.V. DRINK.

I know this sounds really disgusting, and trust me when I say that it definitely is. Even though this is gross, if you mix 1 to 2 teaspoons of apple cider vinegar with 8 ounces of water and drink it, you will eventually begin to notice that your symptoms will begin to go away. This is a very popular treatment for many conditions including acid reflux, just so you know.

Although it's not the most known home remedy for yeast infections, apple cider vinegar can still provide you with relief. I recommend taking a bath with it, because the taste can be pretty foul. If you're going to try to treat yourself internally, there is always yogurt. Yogurt is probably one of the most popular home remedies available.

CHAPTER 8: GOUT PAIN

Apple cider vinegar can be used externally and/or taken internally to help reduce gout pain and inflammation. In this chapter, you'll discover why this type of vinegar can help to alleviate the symptoms of gout and how to use it.

Today, more than ever, gout is affecting more and more people across the globe, who are generally treating their condition with drugs. But since the drugs used for gout today have many side effects, some rather serious in nature, gout sufferers are increasingly seeking out natural ways to treat their affliction.

BENEFITS OF APPLE CIDER VINEGAR

There are many natural remedies for gout out there, but one of the popular ones is apple cider vinegar. Apple cider vinegar has been used since antiquity as a natural home remedy for a whole range of health issues, including gout.

But it must be raw apple cider vinegar that hasn't been distilled or pasteurized. It may be hard to get in most supermarkets, but you should get this special vinegar in health food stores or other speciality stores. You should be able to see a good deal of sediment -- known a the 'mother' -- on the bottom of the bottle.

It is believed that when taken as a drink, this type of cider changes the pH of the blood which is one way to help alleviate high uric acid levels. And when applied externally to the location of the gout, it can help to reduce swelling and relieve the associated pain.

HOW TO DRINK APPLE CIDER VINEGAR FOR GOUT

Mix 2 to 3 teaspoons of vinegar into a large glass of water. Drink such a glass 2 or 3 times daily. Many people can drink it this way, the taste isn't a problem for them. However, if you wish to you can add 2 teaspoons of honey to help the taste.

HOW TO USE APPLE CIDER VINEGAR TOPICALLY

The basic ratio for this application is 1/2 (half) a cup of the vinegar to 3 cups of hot water. But because you are going to immerse the gouty joint in the liquid you'll probably need to make up more. Just stick to the ratio.

For example, to soak your foot, add 2 cups to 12 cups of hot water. Make sure that you test the temperature of the water before immersing your foot or other part of the body where the gout is.

Raw apple cider vinegar is only one of a range of home remedies available to you to treat gout. Other popular remedies are things like, certain fruits and vegetables, herbal remedies, supplements, making particular changes to your diet, some lifestyle adjustments, natural physical medicine, and so on.

CHAPTER 9: AS A NATURAL CLEANING AGENT

Apple cider vinegar is another wonderful natural cleaning agent. It has so many purposes, both in cooking and for household use that this is a definite must have item around the house. You will also save a tremendous amount of money.

This little natural cleaner has been used to clean homes for 10,000 years. It has also been used to promote health and as a beauty enhancer for that amount of time as well. Apple cider vinegar can clean virtually anything, inside and out.

A great solution to remove carpet stains. This includes both pet stains and food stains. Try adding it to your dishwasher and see how much cleaner your dishes come out. It will also treat hard water spots with ease. Add it to your laundry to remove stains there.

It will also brighten clothes and keep them from looking dingy and faded. It will help set any dyes that you might ad as well and you can add it to the rinse cycle and your clothes will be rinsed more thoroughly.

Some people may be concerned about the smell it may leave but all you will be left with is the smell of clean, fresh clothes, no vinegar smell to be found.

A tough spot to clean as always been the grease stained oven and the microwave as well. Keep these items grease and grime free. Removing soap scum from showers, tile, and faucets will be a thing of ease with the help of apple cider vinegar.

Use it to clean floors, counter tops, cabinets, and walls without worrying about if it is going to damage these surfaces or not. It can be used on virtually any hard surface. No need to use a separate disinfectant as apple cider vinegar will conquer that as well.

The uses for apple cider vinegar are endless. Try it on your trashcan, in your bathroom, and kitchen. Have troubled pet areas, it will work there too.

Doorknobs can be one of the leading causes of spreading germs and with a simple wipe down with apple cider vinegar you can eliminate any and all germs. Counter tops and laundry rooms can also benefit from this economical cleaning agent.

Apple cider vinegar is a spectacular general cleaning agent. It can be used on your windows, glass and mirrors, leaving a streak free finish and a shine that you will surely love. This is easy to mix, add one half cup of apple cider vinegar to one half cup of water and you will have a cleaner ready in minutes.

For stubborn stains, such as in the toilet, you can use the apple cider vinegar in full strength. Try to use as little of the cleaning agent as possible and then dry the area with a paper towel. Do not leave excess cleaner on the floor or it can cause damage to your flooring.

There are just so many uses for apple cider vinegar. Whether you are health conscious about the environment or you are looking to save money, this is definitely a great alternative for you household cleaning needs.

CHAPTER 10: ARTHRITIS

Using apple cider vinegar for arthritis is something that has been done for centuries. There are many reasons for this that you should be aware of. Apple cider vinegar actually has many medicinal benefits and relieving arthritis pain is one of them.

One thing to know about arthritis is that it can be characterized by the formation of crystallized uric acid around the joints. The use of apple cider vinegar is recommended to break down these crystals.

This is done by the malic acid that is one of the active compounds of this type of vinegar. The acid will break down the crystals so they can pass out of the body. It should be noted that this does not prevent them from forming.

Inflammation is something that people with arthritis also suffer from. This type of vinegar can help with this as well because it is a natural antioxidant. The antioxidant properties will reduce the inflammation around the joints.

Additionally it is thought that this reduction will help to slow the progress of the condition. Pain relief is also something that this vinegar can help with. The malic and acetic acids in the vinegar also help the body fight infections.

HOW TO USE APPLE CIDER VINEGAR TO FIGHT ARTHRITIS PAIN

There are two common ways in which people can administer apple cider vinegar for arthritis. One is through a compress. To do this, you will heat a solution of one part apple cider vinegar to six parts water. When the mixture is hot to the touch then take it off the heat and soak a cloth in it. Ring out the excess and put it onto aching joints.

Another way to administer this vinegar is as a tonic. Many people take a tablespoon two times a day. It is possible to take this vinegar straight if you do not mind the taste. You could also mix a tablespoon full into a glass of water and have it that way or you can make a tea with a teaspoon of natural honey.

You can't go wrong trying apple cider vinegar for arthritis. The cost of this natural remedy is minimal and the benefits are too numerous to mention. Also buy the brand that has organic raw unfiltered apples to get the best results.

CHAPTER 11: AS A THRUSH REMEDY

Apple cider vinegar is a known home remedy for thrush. Many sufferers who are fed up trying to eliminate their thrush through the usual topical creams and pessaries etc., have turned to natural remedies like apple cider vinegar.

Thrush (also called yeast infection) is an infection caused by the overgrow of a yeast-like fungus called Candida Albicans. A majority of women sufferers have vaginal thrush. Here you'll discover how to use apple cider vinegar for vaginal thrush.

Apple cider vinegar has successfully been used as a natural remedy for a range of ailments for thousands of years. The trace elements, minerals, enzymes, beneficial bacteria, etc., found in raw apple cider vinegar accounts for its healing properties. And thrush is no exception.

But your have to make sure that it is raw, un-distilled and unpasteurized, with no additives or preservatives. You may get it from some grocery stores or supermarkets, but your best bet is your local health food store. Here's how to use it...

As a drink, mix two teaspoons of apple cider vinegar in a glass of water. Drink three times a day. This will help to control the Candida Albicans fungi in your gut.

As a topical medication you can douche with it. Just add two tablespoons of vinegar to two quarts of warm water and gently douche using a cotton pad. Do this twice a day. Stop when the symptoms disappear. The vinegar helps to re-balance your vaginal pH (acidity), thus helping to check the growth of the Candida fungi there.

Many women prefer to bathe. To a warm, low bath add two cups of apple cider vinegar and sit in the bath for around twenty minutes or so. Open the lips of the vagina so that the warm solution can get at the infection better. If you can repeat twice a day until the thrush symptoms go away.

Apple cider vinegar is a very popular home remedy for thrush. But it is only one of many home remedies for thrush in use today. What women have found is that some work better than others, and, what might work for one person might not work for another.

And there are other conflicting factors to consider. For example some of the things that can help the Candida fungi overgrow are things like antibiotic overuse, bad diet, steroids, a compromised immune system, weight issues, drug taking, diabetes, etc. You'll need to factor in all these things to achieve a permanent cure for your thrush.

CHAPTER 12: TREATMENT FOR CELLULITE

Cellulite is the fat deposited beneath the skin surface around the hips, buttocks and thighs. Women of all races are afflicted by cellulite. It is seen mostly in obese women but does not exclusively spare lean women. Though cellulite per say is not indicative of any disease, it is often a cause of concern for cosmetic reasons.

The skin contains bands of elastic tissue that stretch from the skin to the deeper layers of the muscle tissue. These bands are inelastic and as fat is deposited in the subcutaneous area, the only way for it to move is to bulge out on the skin surface. The strands of connective tissue try to keep the skin in place giving the dimpled effect to the skin.

The formation of cellulite is mainly due to imbalance in fatty acid metabolism. Other factors like lack of physical activity and improper diet are also responsible for cellulite deposition. Another contributory factor for cellulite formation is the poor circulation of blood and lymph which leads to accumulation of toxins in the body.

Many remedies are available for cellulite therapy and natural remedies are favored due to their safety profile. Apple cider vinegar is one of the natural remedies used for the treatment of cellulite which has been known for over two thousand years in weight loss therapies.

WHAT IS APPLE CIDER VINEGAR?

Natural Apple Cider Vinegar (ACV) is made by crushing fresh, organically grown apples and allowing them to mature in wooden barrels. This boosts natural fermentation and allows the vinegar to mature.

It is an effective natural bacteria-fighting agent that contains many vital minerals and trace elements such as potassium, calcium, magnesium, phosphorous, chlorine, sodium, sulfur, copper, iron, silicon and fluorine that are vital for a healthy body.

ROLE OF APPLE CIDER VINEGAR IN CELLULITE THERAPY

- Apple cider vinegar strengthens the immune system and cures many infections. It also increases the body's metabolic rate and promotes thermogenesis.

- Due to the increased basal metabolic rate there is increased burning of fat which in turn balances cholesterol and causes weight loss.

- Other micronutrients present in apple cider vinegar like vitamin B6 and lecithin also contribute to weight loss. Since weight control is an essential aspect of cellulite therapy apple cider vinegar becomes extremely useful.

- Apple cider vinegar also helps in getting rid of the excess of fluids accumulated in the body by helping improve the circulation of blood.

- It is also known to curb the appetite.

- Apple cider vinegar is available for use as capsules or liquid . The capsules can be taken as two per day and can be increased to three doses a day if required. The liquid form can be used as two spoonfuls in a glass of water to be taken before every meal.

CHAPTER 13: ATHLETES FOOT

Apple cider vinegar may be the best natural remedy for athlete's foot. It is the ability of this type of vinegar to destroy fungal infections that makes it an ideal natural remedy for athlete's foot fungus.

Not only is it considerably less expensive than prescription drugs and even over the counter medications, pure apple cider vinegar relieves the itching that is caused by athlete's foot making it a gentle, all natural answer to this common and painful problem. And best of all, you may already have it in your cupboard.

Athlete's foot is a well-known, persistent ailment caused by fungal growth on the feet. This type of infection occurs when the highly contagious tinea pedis fungus contacts the skin. Often the most affected area of the foot is between the toes, where it is especially warm and moist; however, it may also spread to the rest of the foot.

When athlete's foot fungus is given an opportunity to develop, it may first result in an itchy red rash, typically beginning between the fourth and fifth toe. If the infection is not remedied, the skin may become soft and extremely sensitive to the touch.

In the most severe cases, the edges of the afflicted area will become white and the skin can peel away, creating a milky discharge.

To combat this unfortunate condition, people have turned time and again to apple cider vinegar. This type of vinegar is made from the liquid extracted from crushed apples. Sugar and yeast are added to encourage fermentation, which turns the sugars into alcohol.

It is in the second fermentation process when acetic acid-forming bacteria transform the alcohol into vinegar.

This acidic product can be used to treat feet that have become raw, cracked, and damaged by the fungus that causes athlete's foot. Not only does it relieve the persistent itch that comes with the condition, it also has been reported to rid the body of the fungus that causes the condition. It may not have the most desirable odor, but the relief that is immediately felt as sore feet contact the vinegar will surely be worth it.

An apple cider vinegar foot soak is an effective way to fight athlete's foot fungus. Simply mix one part pure all natural apple cider vinegar with one part warm water and soak for 20 minutes. Feet should be cleaned with a gentle soap both before and after the treatment.

It is necessary to make sure that the feet are thoroughly dried after the treatment to prevent the fungus from spreading in a moist environment. If necessary, it is permissible to use this method of treatment twice daily. Depending upon the severity of the condition, the feet should be rid of the fungus within one to two weeks of regular home treatments.

For less severe cases of athlete's foot fungus, use a washcloth or cotton ball soaked in apple cider vinegar. Gently rub the cloth over the affected areas. This treatment works especially well for children who may not be willing to sit for a foot soak as the combination of the vinegar and the rubbing of the washcloth allow instant relief from the itchiness caused by the fungus.

It is wise to take some common sense precautions to lessen your exposure to the fungus as preventing athlete's foot fungus is typically much easier than curing it, it. The most important step you can take is to keep the feet dry, especially between the toes.

Ensure that the environment in your socks is inhospitable to fungal growth. Socks that are made of cotton, wool, or other natural materials allow feet to breathe and remain dry.

If your feet commonly sweat, see that your socks remain clean and dry, even if this means changing socks during the day. Choose shoes that are well ventilated and give them a chance to dry out before wearing them again.

It is also important to reduce the risk of exposure by wearing waterproof sandals or shoes in public showers, locker rooms, and any other warm damp place that may host tinea pedis. Taking proper care of your feet and treating them with all natural apple cider vinegar should ensure that the athlete's foot fungus clears up and does not return.

CHAPTER 14: FIBROIDS

There is a lot of talk about fibroids and apple cider vinegar (ACV) and how ACV can help to shrink fibroids naturally. ACV is one of the most commonly recommended natural remedies for many diseases and conditions.

One of the reasons it is a common natural remedy is because it is commonly available in most kitchens, is relatively inexpensive and there are little to no side effects. Despite there being little if any scientific research to support the many health claims of using ACV, this is still a common natural remedy.

As a natural remedy, many people tout the benefits of ACV for a variety of ailments such as diabetes, weight loss, heartburn, psoriasis, dry skin, dry scalp, dry hair, constipation, high cholesterol, nail and ear fungus, arthritis, dandruff, deodorant, kidney stones, warts, jock itch, yeast infection, etc.

While there is little to no scientific proof that ACV may work for many of these ailments, you can find many positive testimonials from people who have used ACV to treat any number of ailments.

One thing to remember about scientific research as it relates to many natural remedies is that there is no incentive for vast amounts of money to be spent on researching remedies such as ACV because it will not be possible to patent ACV since it is readily available.

FIBROIDS AND APPLE CIDER VINEGAR

The acidic nature of ACV may explain its effectiveness against many ailments and why it is considered antibacterial, antifungal and antiviral but it also contains various vitamins and minerals that our bodies need as well as enzymes and very important anti-inflammatory properties all of which can help to fight various ailments.

Many Eastern practitioners believe that sickness and disease including fibroids are caused by an acidic nature in the body and helping the body become more alkaline can help to fight off various diseases and conditions and create a healthier body.

It is very important to note that while the acidic nature of ACV is touted for the healing properties when used topically, when taken internally, ACV actually has an alkaline effect in the body by helping to raise the pH level from an acidic one to a more alkaline one which can help the body become healthier.

Toxins in the body can also increase the risk of developing various diseases and conditions including the development of fibroid tumors. Another of the benefits of ACV is that it helps to detoxify the body.

Being overweight is another risk factor for fibroid development and ACV can help with weight loss which indirectly helps to fight off various weight related diseases and conditions including fibroids.

These health benefits and many more related to ACV is why many women with fibroids commonly tout its ability to shrink fibroids naturally even in the absence of scientific proof.

HOW TO USE APPLE CIDER VINEGAR FOR FIBROIDS

There isn't a set dosage but many women take one tablespoon or two teaspoons of ACV per day. Because consuming neat ACV (undiluted) can wear at the tooth enamel as well as cause burns to the sensitive areas of the throat and mouth, it is recommended to mix it in a liquid.

Most people commonly mix ACV with about 8 ounces of water, tea or milk (soy, almond milk, etc, are better than dairy milk especially for those with fibroids).

Another precaution with ACV is to stay away from ACV supplements because some studies have shown that these supplements can permanently damage the tissue in the esophagus.

BEST APPLE CIDER VINEGAR FOR FIBROIDS

The first recommendation is to of course use ACV and not other types of vinegar (e.g. white vinegar) because ACV is made from apples which is why it contains most of the vitamins, minerals and trace minerals that our bodies need to be healthy. Other types of vinegar such as white vinegar do not contain a lot of these properties.

Another point to remember is that there are varying processes that are used to make ACV many of which can eliminate most of the beneficial properties of ACV. This is why most of those sold in grocery stores should be avoided for internal use because they are lacking in healthful properties.

The best apple cider vinegar to use as a natural remedy is that which is made from organic apples, that is raw, unfiltered and fermented using traditional methods (unpasteurized). It should also state that it includes the "mother" which is where most of the healthful properties of apple cider vinegar reside.

CHAPTER 15: TYPE 2 DIABETES

Apple cider vinegar has been used for many years by people of all cultures and offers a broad range of significant benefits. Let us look at three benefits you should know about...

1. *Blood Sugar Control. The first major benefit you can expect to receive from using apple cider vinegar is stabilized blood sugar levels. For anyone who is experiencing Type 2 diabetes, this is a benefit you will want to take note of.*

Mixing one tablespoon of apple cider vinegar into a cup of water is an excellent way to help reduce the spike in blood sugar you would experience after consuming a carbohydrate rich meal.

2. *PH Balancer. Next, apple cider vinegar is also an excellent way to help balance out your pH levels, ensuring they are normal and within a healthy range.*

If you are someone who consumes a high amount of meat in your diet plan, chances are you are currently more acidic than what is considered to be healthy.

A high protein diet does have this effect, so unless you are making a conscious effort to include a wide variety of fresh fruits and vegetables into your diet each day, you could be in for some unwanted side effects.

These might include feelings of…

Fatigue,

Dizziness,

Having trouble concentrating, as well as

A rapid heart rate or changes in blood pressure.

Despite the fact it is acidic, apple cider vinegar will become more alkaline once it enters your system. Therefore, it can help take you away from that highly acidic state, making you healthier overall.

3. *Allergy Control. Finally, apple cider vinegar may just assist you in combating seasonal allergies as well. It can help to eliminate the mucus in your sinuses, making it easier to breathe.*

If you are someone who typically relies on over-the-counter allergy medication, you may know these often come with the side effect of causing one to be exceptionally drowsy. Try a natural treatment, and you may be able to side-step that.

As you can see, there are several reasons to include apple cider vinegar in your daily diet plan, and these few reasons are just the tip of the iceberg. There are many more great uses for apple cider vinegar, so do some of your research and make sure you are not missing out on some of the benefits associated with this powerful ingredient.

Although managing your disease can be very challenging, Type 2 diabetes is not a condition you must just live with. You can make simple changes to your daily routine and lower both your weight and your blood sugar levels. Hang in there, the longer you do it, the easier it gets.

CHAPTER 16: HEARTBURN

Apple cider vinegar is a folk remedy for getting rid of heartburn. In fact, it is the TOP folk remedy for heartburn and acid reflux.

RECIPE FOR RELIEF

Taking apple cider vinegar for heartburn relief is quite simple. Simply stir 2 Tablespoons of apple cider vinegar into 1/2 cup of water or apple juice. Drink this immediately after each meal. If your problem is acid reflux, and you have just had a heavy meal, increase the amount of apple cider vinegar and decrease the amount of water or juice.

Another option is to mix a "cocktail" of the following:

- 1 quart apple juice

- 1 pint purple grape juice

- 1/2 cup apple cider vinegar

Drink 1/2 cup after every meal for heartburn relief.

Recipes that use apple cider vinegar for getting rid of heartburn vary greatly. This is because individual bodies also vary greatly. Try different amounts of apple cider vinegar until you find what works for you.

Some people have found that one brand or another works better for them. Again, the difference is due to the variations in physical makeup.

HOW APPLE CIDER VINEGAR REMEDIES HEARTBURN

Little research has been done on the effectiveness of apple cider vinegar for heartburn relief. Consequently, it is difficult to say how apple cider vinegar remedies heartburn.

It appears that the acid content in vinegar somehow tells the stomach to stop producing more acid. Perhaps, in that way, apple cider vinegar is like the prescription medications that "shut down" the stomach's acid pumps to stop heartburn.

Apple cider vinegar does not taste good to most people. Because of that, some have tried eating a few slices of apple after a meal, and have gotten rid of heartburn that way. Not every apple works for heartburn, though. Some stick to green apples such as Granny Smith.

Others recommend Jonagold apples for heartburn relief. Some recommend eating a few slices of Jonagold apple with a couple of dill pickle spears. It's apple cider vinegar for heartburn without resorting to basic vinegar.

CHAPTER 17: BACTERIAL VAGIOSIS

BV, or bacterial vagiosis, is not a fun condition. It can cause both the inside and outside of your vagina to become swollen, painful and itchy. It can also cause discharge and unpleasant smells to come from your vagina.

Meanwhile, you may also find yourself experiencing cramps, bloating or even bleeding associated with your BV. That can really make you miserable and it can certainly kill your sex life. So, it's a condition that most women are in a hurry to cure.

KILLING THE BACTERIA:

The traditional medical way to cure BV, which is a bacterial infection, is to kill off the offending bacteria. Your doctor might suggest that you do that by taking antibiotics.

However, antibiotics will kill all bacteria and the thing that many women don't understand is that a woman's vagina is supposed to contain healthy bacteria, which protect it.

ALTERING THE BALANCE:

The reason that apple cider vinegar works so well as a treatment for BV is that it is slightly acidic. Therefore, it has the power to alter the pH balance of your vagina just enough to allow good bacteria to stay healthy and keep bad bacteria from growing.

So, you can slightly adjust your vaginal environment, rather than obliterating all of the bacteria with antibiotics.

A VINEGAR BATH:

If you're going to use apple cider vinegar to relieve BV symptoms, one easy way to do that is to take an apple cider vinegar bath. Start by running a warm, shallow bath. Then, mix in about half to a whole cup of the vinegar with the bath water. Be careful not to add too much vinegar because that could cause a severe burning sensation when you sit down in the tub.

An apple cider vinegar bath can be useful, but you shouldn't do it too often. Remember that you just want to restore the balance in your vagina. Tipping the scales too far in the other direction might just make your problems worse.

A VINEGAR DOUCHE:

Like a vinegar bath, a vinegar douche should be quite diluted. A teaspoon of apple cider vinegar in two cups of water should be fine. Also, as with a vinegar bath, you shouldn't douche too often. Once a day is quite enough to get the job done.

DRINKING VINEGAR:

Drinking a little apple cider vinegar is a good way to prevent BV, although it may not be as helpful as a bath or douche in terms of curing an existing BV outbreak.

However, using apple cider vinegar for BV relief, especially if you plan to drink it, should be done with care. Since it is slightly acidic, you don't need or want large quantities of it in your body. So, use it in moderation and you should find that it can bring you some much needed BV relief.

CONCLUSION

Recently apple cider vinegar has been deemed a very helpful health elixir. What once used to be considered folk remedies using this is now backed by scientific research indicating its helpful effects. The primary ingredient is acetic acid. Vinegars also have other acids, vitamins, mineral salts and amino acids.

Vinegar is a product of the process of fermentation by which sugars in a food are broken down by bacteria in yeast. In the second stage of fermentation the alcohol ferments further and we get vinegar.Specifically, apple cider vinegar comes from crushed apples.

Because of the widespread claims that it can promote health benefits, scientific evidence has been evaluated and has shown that this indeed is true.

The popularity of apple cider vinegar continues to this day. And the best part is that it is readily available at your local supermarket.

TRY APPLE CIDER VINEGAR TODAY!

www.ingramcontent.com/pod-product-compliance
Lightning Source LLC
Chambersburg PA
CBHW070828260726
48654CB00024B/551